CONGESTIVE HEART FAILURE COOKBOOK

Simple and Easy-to-make delicious and Nutritious Low Fat and Low Sodium Recipes to Reduce Blood Pressure and Boost Heart Health

Dr. Mary D. Torres

Copyright 2023 by Dr. Mary D. Torres

All rights reserved.

This copyright applies to the entire contents of this cookbook, including but not limited to text, recipes, illustrations, photographs, and design. No part of this cookbook may be reproduced, distributed, or transmitted in any form or by any means, including photocopying, recording, or other electronic or mechanical methods, without the prior written permission of the copyright holder, except for brief quotations embodied in critical reviews and certain other non-commercial uses permitted by copyright law.

DISCLAIMER

The Congestive Heart Failure Cookbook is a collection of recipes and dietary guidelines intended to support individuals managing congestive heart failure. While every effort has been made to ensure the accuracy and reliability of the information presented, it is essential to note that this cookbook is not a substitute for professional medical advice, diagnosis, or treatment.

Readers are strongly advised to consult with a qualified healthcare professional or registered dietitian before making significant changes to their diet, especially if they are managing specific medical conditions, such as congestive heart failure. The recipes and nutritional information provided in this cookbook are general recommendations and may not be suitable for everyone.

Individuals with food allergies, sensitivities, or dietary restrictions should exercise caution and carefully review the ingredient lists, considering their unique health circumstances. The authors, publishers, and contributors of this cookbook cannot be held responsible for any adverse effects, reactions, or consequences resulting from the use of the recipes or information contained herein.

The goal of this cookbook is to provide inspiration and guidance for crafting heart-healthy meals, but individual health requirements may vary.

By using this cookbook, readers acknowledge and agree to the terms of this disclaimer.

TABLE OF CONTENTS

INTRODUCTION... **5**

CHAPTER 1: OVERVIEW OF CONGESTIVE HEART FAILURE **7**

What is Congestive Heart Failure? 7

Types of Congestive Heart Failure 7

Symptoms of Congestive Heart Failure 10

Importance of Low Fat and Low Sodium Diet for Heart Health 12

Importance of Diet in Managing Heart Health.....................15

CHAPTER 2: BREAKFAST TO KICKSTART YOUR DAY **19**

CHAPTER 3: LUNCH FOR SUSTAINED ENERGY33

CHAPTER 4: SOUP AND SALAD RECIPES........ **49**

CHAPTER 5: HEART FRIENDLY DESERTS...... **62**

CHAPTER 6: NOURISHING DINNER FOR HEART HEALTH.. **72**

CHAPTER 7: BEVERAGES FOR HYDRATION . **83**

CHAPTER 8: SNACKS AND APPETIZERS......... **94**

CONCLUSION **105**

7-WEEK MEAL PLANNING 107

INTRODUCTION

John, my cousin has been living with congestive heart failure for several years. He has always been a food lover, but after his diagnosis, he struggled to find delicious and satisfying meals that were also low in fat and sodium. That's when he discovered this "Congestive Heart Failure Cookbook."

At first, John was skeptical. He had tried other heart-healthy cookbooks in the past, but the recipes were often bland and unappetizing. However, after flipping through the pages of this cookbook, he was pleasantly surprised. The recipes looked delicious and easy to make, and the ingredients were readily available at his local grocery store.

John started with the breakfast section and made the low-fat oatmeal with fresh berries. He was amazed at how flavorful and satisfying it was, despite being low in fat and sodium. He then moved on to the soups and salads section and made the heart-healthy minestrone soup. Again, he was impressed with how delicious it was, and he loved that it was packed with vegetables and fiber.

Over the next few weeks, John continued to try new recipes from the cookbook. He made the baked lemon herb chicken, the quinoa and black bean stuffed peppers, and the dark chocolate avocado mousse. Each recipe was a hit, and John was thrilled to have found a cookbook that allowed him to enjoy delicious meals while also managing his congestive heart failure.

Since incorporating the recipes from this cookbook into his diet, John has noticed a significant improvement in his health. His blood pressure has decreased, and he has more energy and stamina. He feels more in control of his condition and is grateful for the positive impact that proper dieting has had on his life.

Above all, this **"Congestive Heart Failure Cookbook"** has been a game-changer for John and many others living with this condition. It offers delicious and nutritious recipes that are easy to make and satisfying to eat. By simply following the guidelines and recipes in this cookbook, anyone with congestive heart failure can improve their health and quality of life.

CHAPTER 1: OVERVIEW OF CONGESTIVE HEART FAILURE

What is Congestive Heart Failure?

Congestive heart failure (CHF) is a chronic medical condition in which the heart is unable to pump blood effectively, leading to an inadequate supply of oxygen and nutrients to the body's tissues. This condition does not mean that the heart has completely stopped working, but rather that it is struggling to meet the body's demands.

In a healthy heart, blood is pumped out to the body through the left ventricle, supplying oxygen and nutrients. In congestive heart failure, the heart's pumping ability weakens, causing blood to move through the heart and the body at a slower rate. This leads to a backlog of blood in the vessels, resulting in congestion or fluid buildup in various parts of the body, particularly the lungs and extremities.

Types of Congestive Heart Failure

Heart failure is a serious condition, and it can be classified into different types based on various factors, including the part of the heart affected or the underlying causes.

The two main types of heart failure are systolic heart failure and diastolic heart failure. Additionally, heart failure can be categorized as left-sided or right-sided, depending on which side of the heart is primarily affected.

Systolic Heart Failure:

In systolic heart failure, the heart's left ventricle becomes weakened and is unable to contract effectively during each heartbeat. This results in a reduced ejection fraction, which is the amount of blood pumped out of the heart with each contraction. Systolic heart failure is often referred to as heart failure with reduced ejection fraction (HFrEF).

Diastolic Heart Failure:

Diastolic heart failure happens when the left ventricle becomes stiff and less compliant, impairing its ability to relax and fill with blood during the resting phase between heartbeats. This often leads to a reduced capacity to accommodate blood. Diastolic heart failure is sometimes known as heart failure with preserved ejection fraction (HFpEF).

Left-Sided Heart Failure:

Left-sided heart failure is the most common type. It can be further divided into systolic and diastolic heart failure. This means that when the left side of the heart fails, blood backs up into the lungs, causing symptoms like shortness of breath and fluid retention.

Right-Sided Heart Failure:

Right-sided heart failure usually occurs as a result of left-sided heart failure. When the left ventricle is unable to pump blood effectively, it can lead to a backup of blood in the veins returning to the right side of the heart. This, in turn, causes the right side of the heart to work harder, eventually leading to right-sided heart failure. Symptoms usually include swelling in the legs and abdomen.

Acute and Chronic Heart Failure:

Heart failure can be classified based on its duration. Acute heart failure refers to a sudden onset or worsening of symptoms and may require immediate medical attention. Chronic heart failure, on the other hand, develops over time and persists as an ongoing condition. Many individuals with chronic heart failure experience periods of acute exacerbation.

Symptoms of Congestive Heart Failure

Congestive heart failure (CHF) can manifest a variety of symptoms, and their severity may vary from person to person. Some common symptoms of congestive heart failure include:

Shortness of Breath (Dyspnea):

Difficulty breathing, especially during physical activity or when lying down.

Persistent Coughing:

A chronic cough, often accompanied by white or pink-tinged phlegm. This can be a result of fluid buildup in the lungs.

Fatigue and Weakness:

Persistent tiredness and a sense of weakness, even with minimal exertion.

Swelling (Edema):

Swelling in the legs, ankles, or abdomen due to the accumulation of fluid. This is a common sign of fluid retention.

Rapid or Irregular Heartbeat:

Palpitations, rapid heartbeat, or irregular heart rhythms (arrhythmias).

Reduced Exercise Tolerance:

Inability to engage in physical activities or exercise to the same extent as before.

Increased Urination at Night:

Frequent or consistent urination, particularly at night, as the body tries to eliminate excess fluid.

Sudden Weight Gain:

Unexplained weight gain over a short period, often due to fluid retention.

Loss of Appetite and Nausea:

A decreased desire to eat, possibly accompanied by nausea.

Difficulty Concentrating or Confusion:

Impaired cognitive function, difficulty concentrating, or confusion may occur due to reduced blood flow to the brain.

Chest Pain or Discomfort:

While chest pain is not always present, it can occur and may be a sign of reduced blood flow to the heart muscle.

Importance of Low Fat and Low Sodium Diet for Heart Health

Starting and adopting a low-fat and low-sodium diet is paramount for maintaining heart health and preventing cardiovascular conditions. To understand better, below are some of the importance of these dietary choices:

1. Reducing Risk of Heart Disease:

A diet low in saturated and trans fats helps lower levels of harmful LDL cholesterol in the bloodstream. Increased LDL cholesterol is a significant risk factor for heart disease and atherosclerosis, where arteries become narrowed and hardened.

2. Managing Blood Pressure:

High sodium intake is linked to high blood pressure (hypertension), In fact, this is a leading cause of heart disease. A low-sodium diet helps regulate blood pressure by minimizing fluid retention and reducing the strain on the heart.

3. Preventing Congestive Heart Failure:

Congestive heart failure occurs when the heart is unable to pump blood effectively. By controlling sodium intake and maintaining a diet low in saturated fats, the risk of developing conditions that contribute to heart failure, such as hypertension and coronary artery disease is reduced.

4. Supporting Weight Management:

A low-fat diet is instrumental in weight management, as fat is calorie-dense. Excess weight can strain the heart, leading to conditions like heart disease and diabetes. Additionally, maintaining a healthy weight contributes to overall cardiovascular well-being.

5. Improving Cholesterol Levels:

Low-fat diets, especially those emphasizing healthy fats like omega-3 fatty acids, can improve cholesterol profiles. It is best to reduce LDL cholesterol and increase HDL cholesterol, the risk of arterial plaque formation decreases.

6. Enhancing Vascular Function:

Diets rich in fruits, vegetables, and whole grains, which are typically low in fat and sodium provide essential nutrients and antioxidants that promote vascular health. Healthy blood vessels contribute to efficient blood flow and reduce the risk of clot formation.

7. Regulating Blood Sugar Levels:

Low-fat and low-sodium diets can positively impact blood sugar levels and reduce the risk of diabetes. Diabetes is a significant risk factor for heart disease, making blood sugar control crucial for heart health.

8. Encouraging Heart-Healthy Nutrient Intake:

Adopting a low-fat and low-sodium diet often involves choosing nutrient-dense foods. This ensures an adequate intake of vitamins, minerals, and fiber, which are essential for overall cardiovascular and metabolic health.

9. Minimizing Fluid Retention:

Low-sodium intake helps prevent fluid retention, help alleviate stress on the heart and reducing the likelihood of conditions like edema.

10. Promoting Overall Well-Being:

Adopting heart-healthy dietary habits contributes to overall well-being, fostering energy, vitality, and a reduced risk of chronic diseases beyond cardiovascular conditions.

Importance of Diet in Managing Heart Health

Diet plays a pivotal role in managing heart health, influencing various factors that contribute to cardiovascular well-being. Here are key aspects highlighting the importance of diet in maintaining heart health:

Cholesterol Control:

A heart-healthy diet helps manage cholesterol levels, particularly by reducing the intake of saturated and trans fats. Lowering LDL (low-density lipoprotein) cholesterol, often termed "bad" cholesterol, and increasing HDL (high-density lipoprotein) cholesterol, known as "good" cholesterol, are critical for preventing atherosclerosis and maintaining clear arteries.

Blood Pressure Regulation:

Adopting a diet low in sodium and rich in potassium, magnesium, and fiber helps regulate and manage blood pressure. High blood pressure is a major risk factor for heart disease, stroke, and other cardiovascular complications.

Weight Management:

Maintaining a healthy weight is essential for heart health. A balanced diet that includes nutrient-dense foods promotes weight management by providing necessary nutrients without excessive calories. Obesity is a significant risk factor for heart disease and related conditions.

Diabetes Prevention and Management:

A heart-healthy diet can help prevent and manage diabetes; a condition closely linked to cardiovascular disease. Controlling blood sugar levels through dietary choices minimizes the risk of diabetic complications affecting the heart and blood vessels.

Reducing Inflammation:

Certain foods, such as fruits, vegetables, and omega-3 fatty acids, possess anti-inflammatory properties. Chronic inflammation is associated with heart disease, and an anti-inflammatory diet can contribute to overall cardiovascular health.

Promoting Healthy Fats:

Including sources of healthy fats, such as monounsaturated and polyunsaturated fats found in olive oil, avocados, and fatty fish, supports heart health. These fats can improve cholesterol profiles and reduce the risk of coronary artery disease.

Encouraging Fiber Intake:

A diet rich in fiber from fruits, vegetables, whole grains, and legumes helps lower cholesterol levels, regulate blood sugar, and promote satiety. Fiber also contributes to digestive health and weight management.

Antioxidant Protection:

Antioxidant-rich foods, including berries, nuts, and leafy greens, protect the heart by neutralizing free radicals and reducing oxidative stress. This can help prevent damage to blood vessels and lower the risk of heart disease.

Balancing Macronutrients:

Achieving a balance of carbohydrates, proteins, and fats in the diet ensures optimal energy levels and supports overall health. A well-rounded diet provides the necessary nutrients for the heart to function efficiently.

Heart-Healthy Nutrient Intake:

Consuming foods high in essential nutrients, such as potassium, magnesium, and calcium, contributes to heart health. These nutrients are vital for maintaining proper heart rhythm, blood vessel function, and overall cardiovascular stability.

CHAPTER 2: BREAKFAST TO KICKSTART YOUR DAY

1. **Oatmeal with Fresh Berries:**

Benefits: High-fiber oats with antioxidants from fresh berries.

Ingredients:

Rolled oats

Low-fat milk or water

Fresh berries (strawberries, blueberries)

Honey (optional)

Preparation:

Cook oats with milk or water; top with fresh berries and a drizzle of honey.

2. Whole Wheat Banana Pancakes:

Benefits: Whole grains and potassium from bananas.

Ingredients:

Whole wheat flour

Mashed ripe bananas

Low-fat milk

Baking powder

Preparation:

Mix flour, mashed bananas, milk, and baking powder; cook as pancakes.

3. Greek Yogurt Parfait:

Benefits: Protein-rich Greek yogurt with fiber from fruits and granola.

Ingredients:

Greek yogurt

Mixed berries

Granola (low-sugar)

Almonds, chopped

Preparation:

Layer Greek yogurt with berries, granola, and chopped almonds.

4. **Egg White Veggie Omelets:**

Benefits: High-protein, low-fat omelets with veggies.

Ingredients:

Egg whites

Spinach

Tomatoes, diced

Bell peppers, diced

Feta cheese (optional)

Preparation:

Whisk egg whites; cook with veggies and feta, fold into an omelets.

5. Smoothie Bowl with Spinach and Berries:

Benefits: Antioxidants, fiber, and vitamins in a refreshing bowl.

Ingredients:

Spinach

Mixed berries

Banana

Low-fat yogurt

Chia seeds

Preparation:

Blend spinach, berries, banana, and yogurt; top with chia seeds.

6. Whole Grain Toast with Avocado:

Benefits: Healthy fats and fiber from avocado on whole grain.

Ingredients:

Whole grain bread

Avocado

Cherry tomatoes, sliced

Salt-free seasoning

Preparation:

Toast bread; spread avocado, top with tomatoes and seasoning.

7. Chia Seed Pudding with Mango:

Benefits: Omega-3s and fiber in a delicious pudding.

Ingredients:

Chia seeds

Low-fat milk or almond milk

Mango, diced

Honey (optional)

Preparation:

Mix chia seeds with milk; refrigerate overnight. Top with diced mango and honey.

8. **Cottage Cheese and Pineapple Bowl:**

Benefits: Protein-packed cottage cheese with vitamin C from pineapple.

Ingredients:

Low-fat cottage cheese

Pineapple chunks

Almonds, sliced

Preparation:

Combine cottage cheese with pineapple; sprinkle with sliced almonds.

9. Whole Wheat Banana Muffins:

Benefits: Whole grain goodness with natural sweetness.

Ingredients:

Whole wheat flour

Ripe bananas, mashed

Low-fat yogurt

Baking soda

Preparation:

Mix flour, mashed bananas, yogurt, and baking soda; bake as muffins.

10. Yogurt and Berry Smoothie:

Benefits: Low-fat yogurt with antioxidants from berries.

Ingredients:

Low-fat yogurt

Mixed berries

Banana

Ice cubes

Preparation:

Blend yogurt, berries, banana, and ice cubes until smooth.

11. Low-Sodium Veggie Frittata:

Benefits: Protein and veggies in a flavorful frittata.

Ingredients:

Eggs

Zucchini, diced

Tomatoes, sliced

Low-sodium seasoning

Preparation:

Whisk eggs; cook with veggies and seasoning until set.

12. Peanut Butter Banana Wrap:

Benefits: Protein and potassium in a simple breakfast wrap.

Ingredients:

Whole wheat wrap

Peanut butter (low-sugar)

Sliced banana

Preparation:

Spread peanut butter on the wrap; add sliced banana and fold.

13. Blueberry Almond Chia Pudding:

Benefits: Omega-3s, antioxidants, and fiber in a tasty pudding.

Ingredients:

Chia seeds

Almond milk

Blueberries

Almonds, chopped

Preparation:

Mix chia seeds with almond milk; refrigerate. Top with blueberries and chopped almonds.

14. Cranberry Orange Quinoa Bowl:

Benefits: Quinoa, vitamin C, and antioxidants in a vibrant bowl.

Ingredients:

Cooked quinoa

Dried cranberries

Orange segments

Almonds, sliced

Preparation:

Combine quinoa with cranberries, orange segments, and sliced almonds.

15. Low-Fat Banana Bread:

Benefits: Whole grain banana bread with reduced fat.

Ingredients:

Whole wheat flour

Ripe bananas, mashed, Low-fat yogurt

Baking powder

Preparation:

Mix flour, mashed bananas, yogurt, and baking powder; bake as banana bread.

16. Veggie and Egg Breakfast Burrito:

Benefits: Protein-packed eggs with fiber-rich vegetables.

Ingredients:

Whole wheat tortilla

Eggs, scrambled

Bell peppers, onions, and spinach

Low-sodium salsa

Preparation:

Sauté veggies; add scrambled eggs. Fill tortilla and top with salsa.

17. Peach and Walnut Overnight Oats:

Benefits: Overnight oats with the sweetness of peaches and the crunch of walnuts.

Ingredients:

Rolled oats

Low-fat milk or almond milk

Fresh peach slices

Walnuts, chopped

Preparation:

Mix oats with milk; refrigerate overnight. Top with peach slices and chopped walnuts.

18. Low-Sodium Veggie and Cheese Bagel:

Benefits: Whole grain bagel with veggies and reduced-sodium cheese.

Ingredients:

Whole grain bagel

Low-sodium cream cheese

Tomato slices, cucumber, and red onion

Preparation:

Spread cream cheese on the bagel; top with veggies.

19. Cinnamon Apple Quinoa Porridge:

Benefits: Quinoa porridge with the sweetness of cinnamon apples.

Ingredients:

Cooked quinoa

Apple, diced

Cinnamon

Almond milk

Preparation:

Heat cooked quinoa with diced apples, cinnamon, and almond milk.

20. Low-Fat Mango Banana Smoothie:

Benefits: Tropical smoothie with low-fat yogurt and potassium from mango and banana.

Ingredients:

Low-fat yogurt

Mango, diced

Banana

Ice cubes

Preparation:

Blend yogurt, mango, banana, and ice cubes until smooth

CHAPTER 3: LUNCH FOR SUSTAINED ENERGY

1. Grilled Chicken Salad with Balsamic Vinaigrette:

Description: A refreshing salad with grilled chicken, vibrant veggies, and a tangy balsamic vinaigrette.

Benefits: Lean protein, antioxidants, and heart-healthy fats.

Ingredients:

Grilled chicken breast

Mixed greens

Cherry tomatoes

Cucumber

Avocado

Balsamic vinaigrette

Preparation:

Combine grilled chicken, mixed greens, tomatoes, cucumber, and avocado. Drizzle with balsamic vinaigrette.

2. Vegetarian Quinoa Stir-Fry:

Description: A colorful quinoa stir-fry with a variety of vegetables and flavorful herbs.

Benefits: Plant-based protein, fiber, and essential nutrients.

Ingredients:

Quinoa

Mixed vegetables (bell peppers, broccoli, carrots)

Low-sodium soy sauce

Garlic, minced

Preparation:

Cook quinoa; stir-fry vegetables with garlic and soy sauce. Mix with quinoa.

3. Salmon and Asparagus Foil Packets:

Description: Easy-to-make foil packets with salmon, asparagus, and herbs for a flavorful lunch.

Benefits: Omega-3 fatty acids, vitamins, and minerals.

Ingredients:

Salmon fillets

Asparagus spears

Lemon slices

Fresh dill

Preparation:

Place salmon, asparagus, lemon, and dill in foil packets. Bake until cooked through.

4. **Mediterranean Chickpea Salad:**

Description: A hearty chickpea salad with Mediterranean flavors and a lemon-tahini dressing.

Benefits: Plant-based protein, fiber, and heart-healthy fats.

Ingredients:

Chickpeas

Cherry tomatoes, Cucumber

Kalamata olives, Feta cheese

Lemon-tahini dressing

Preparation:

Combine chickpeas, tomatoes, cucumber, olives, and feta. Drizzle with lemon-tahini dressing.

5. Turkey and Veggie Lettuce Wraps:

Description: Light and satisfying lettuce wraps filled with lean turkey and colorful vegetables.

Benefits: Lean protein, fiber, and a variety of nutrients.

Ingredients:

Ground turkey

Lettuce leaves

Bell peppers, julienned

Carrots, shredded

Hoisin sauce (low-sodium)

Preparation:

Cook ground turkey; fill lettuce leaves with turkey, bell peppers, and carrots. Drizzle with low-sodium hoisin sauce.

6. Sweet Potato and Black Bean Bowl:

Description: A nourishing bowl with roasted sweet potatoes, black beans, and a zesty cilantro-lime dressing.

Benefits: Fiber, antioxidants, and essential vitamins.

Ingredients:

Sweet potatoes, cubed

Black beans

Corn kernels

Red onion, finely chopped

Cilantro-lime dressing

Preparation:

Roast sweet potatoes; mix with black beans, corn, and red onion. Drizzle with cilantro-lime dressing.

7. Lemon Herb Shrimp Skewers:

Description: Grilled shrimp skewers with a zesty lemon-herb marinade.

Benefits: Lean protein, omega-3s, and a burst of citrus flavor.

Ingredients:

Shrimp, peeled and deveined

Lemon juice

Fresh herbs (parsley, thyme)

Garlic, minced

Preparation:

Marinate shrimp in lemon juice, herbs, and garlic. Thread onto skewers and grill.

8. **Cauliflower Fried Rice:**

Description: A low-carb twist on classic fried rice with cauliflower rice, veggies, and lean protein.

Benefits: Low-carb, fiber, and a variety of vegetables.

Ingredients:

Cauliflower rice

Peas and carrots, diced

Eggs, scrambled

Low-sodium soy sauce

Preparation:

Sauté cauliflower rice, peas, carrots, and scrambled eggs. Drizzle with low-sodium soy sauce.

9. Caprese Stuffed Chicken Breast:

Description: Juicy chicken breasts stuffed with tomatoes, mozzarella, and fresh basil.

Benefits: Lean protein, lycopene, and calcium.

Ingredients:

Chicken breasts

Cherry tomatoes, sliced

Fresh mozzarella, sliced

Fresh basil leaves

Preparation:

Cut a pocket in chicken breasts; stuff with tomatoes, mozzarella, and basil. Bake until cooked.

9. Lentil and Vegetable Soup:

Description: A heartwarming soup with lentils, vegetables, and aromatic herbs.

Benefits: Plant-based protein, fiber, and a variety of nutrients.

Ingredients:

Lentils

Carrots, celery, and onions, diced

Low-sodium vegetable broth

Herbs (thyme, rosemary)

Preparation:

Cook lentils; simmer with diced vegetables and herbs in vegetable broth.

11. Tuna and White Bean Salad:

Description: A protein-packed salad with tuna, white beans, and a lemon-olive oil dressing.

Benefits: Omega-3s, fiber, and heart-healthy fats.

Ingredients:

Canned tuna, drained

Cannellini beans

Red onion, finely chopped

Lemon-olive oil dressing

Preparation:

Mix tuna, beans, and red onion. Drizzle with lemon-olive oil dressing.

12. Stuffed Bell Peppers with Quinoa and Turkey:

Description: Bell peppers filled with a wholesome mix of quinoa, lean turkey, and vegetables.

Benefits: Protein, fiber, and a range of vitamins.

Ingredients:

Bell peppers, halved

Ground turkey

Quinoa

Tomatoes, diced

Italian seasoning

Preparation:

Cook quinoa and turkey; mix with tomatoes and Italian seasoning. Fill bell pepper halves and bake.

13. Broccoli and Chicken Stir-Fry:

Description: A quick and nutritious stir-fry with broccoli, chicken, and a savory low-sodium sauce.

Benefits: Lean protein, fiber, and cruciferous vegetables.

Ingredients:

Chicken breast, sliced

Broccoli florets

Low-sodium stir-fry sauce

Brown rice (optional)

Preparation:

Stir-fry chicken and broccoli; add low-sodium stir-fry sauce. Serve over brown rice if desired.

14. Avocado and Black Bean Wrap:

Description: A satisfying wrap with creamy avocado, black beans, and colorful veggies.

Benefits: Healthy fats, fiber, and a variety of nutrients.

Ingredients:

Whole wheat wrap

Black beans, drained and rinsed

Avocado, sliced

Bell peppers, thinly sliced

Cilantro-lime dressing (low-sodium)

Preparation:

Spread black beans on the wrap; add avocado, bell peppers, and drizzle with cilantro-lime dressing.

15. Cucumber and Quinoa Salad with Lemon Dill Dressing:

Description: A refreshing salad with cucumber, quinoa, and a zesty lemon dill dressing.

Benefits: Hydration, protein, and antioxidants.

Ingredients:

Cucumber, diced

Quinoa

Red onion, finely chopped

Lemon dill dressing (low-sodium)

Preparation:

Combine cucumber, quinoa, and red onion. Drizzle with lemon dill dressing.

16. Baked Cod with Lemon and Herbs:

Description: Light and flaky baked cod with a zesty lemon and herb marinade.

Benefits: Lean protein, omega-3s, and fresh flavors.

Ingredients:

Cod fillets

Lemon juice

Fresh herbs (parsley, dill)

Garlic, minced

Preparation:

Marinate cod in lemon juice, herbs, and garlic. Bake until cooked through.

17. Chickpea and Vegetable Curry:

Description: A flavorful chickpea curry with an abundance of vegetables and aromatic spices.

Benefits: Plant-based protein, fiber, and antioxidant-rich spices.

Ingredients:

Chickpeas

Mixed vegetables (cauliflower, peas, carrots)

Curry spices (turmeric, cumin, coriander)

Low-fat coconut milk

Preparation:

Simmer chickpeas and vegetables in a curry spice-infused coconut milk.

18. Spinach and Mushroom Quiche:

Description: A savory quiche filled with nutrient-rich spinach, mushrooms, and a light egg custard.

Benefits: Protein, iron, and vitamins from spinach and mushrooms.

Ingredients:

Pie crust (whole wheat, if available)

Fresh spinach

Mushrooms, sliced

Eggs

Low-fat milk

Preparation:

Sauté spinach and mushrooms; place in a pie crust. Whisk eggs and milk; pour over vegetables. Bake until set.

19. Turkey and Vegetable Kebabs:

Description: Grilled turkey and vegetable kebabs with a savory marinade for a delightful lunch.

Benefits: Lean protein, antioxidants, and a colorful array of veggies.

Ingredients:

Turkey breast, cubed

Bell peppers (various colors), onion, cherry tomatoes

Olive oil, garlic, and herbs

Preparation:

Marinate turkey and vegetables in olive oil, garlic, and herbs. Thread onto skewers and grill.

20. Vegetable and Lentil Stuffed Bell Peppers:

Description: Bell peppers filled with a wholesome mixture of lentils, vegetables, and aromatic spices.

Benefits: Plant-based protein, fiber, and a variety of nutrients.

Ingredients:

Bell peppers, halved

Lentils

Zucchini, tomatoes, onions, diced

Italian seasoning

Preparation:

Cook lentils; mix with diced vegetables and Italian seasoning. Fill bell pepper halves and bake.

CHAPTER 4: SOUP AND SALAD RECIPES

1. Minestrone Soup:

Description: A classic Italian soup with a variety of colorful vegetables, beans, and whole wheat pasta.

Benefits: Fiber, vitamins, and minerals from vegetables; plant-based protein from beans.

Ingredients:

Low-sodium vegetable broth

Tomatoes, diced

Carrots, celery, zucchini, and green beans, chopped

Cannellini beans

Whole wheat pasta

Preparation:

Sauté vegetables, add broth, beans, and pasta. Simmer until vegetables are tender.

2. Greek Salad with Grilled Chicken:

Description: A refreshing Greek salad featuring grilled chicken, tomatoes, cucumbers, olives, and feta.

Benefits: Lean protein from chicken; antioxidants and healthy fats from olives and feta.

Ingredients:

Grilled chicken breast

Cherry tomatoes, halved

Cucumber, diced

Kalamata olives

Feta cheese

Greek dressing (low-sodium)

Preparation:

Toss grilled chicken, tomatoes, cucumber, olives, and feta. Drizzle with low-sodium Greek dressing.

3. Butternut Squash Soup:

Description: Creamy butternut squash soup with a hint of nutmeg, perfect for a warm and comforting meal.

Benefits: Vitamins A and C from butternut squash; low-fat and low-sodium.

Ingredients:

Butternut squash, peeled and cubed

Onion, chopped

Low-sodium vegetable broth

Nutmeg, ground

Preparation:

Sauté onion; add butternut squash and broth. Simmer until squash is tender, then blend until smooth. Season with ground nutmeg.

4. Tuna and White Bean Salad:

Description: A protein-packed salad with tuna, white beans, cherry tomatoes, and a lemon-olive oil dressing.

Benefits: Omega-3s from tuna; plant-based protein from white beans.

Ingredients:

Canned tuna, drained

Cannellini beans

Cherry tomatoes, halved

Red onion, finely chopped

Lemon-olive oil dressing (low-sodium)

Preparation:

Mix tuna, beans, tomatoes, and red onion. Drizzle with low-sodium lemon-olive oil dressing.

5. **Tomato Basil Soup:**

Description: A simple and flavorful tomato basil soup with the goodness of ripe tomatoes and fresh basil.

Benefits: Lycopene from tomatoes; low in fat and sodium.

Ingredients:

Ripe tomatoes, diced

Onion, chopped

Low-sodium vegetable broth

Fresh basil leaves

Preparation:

Sauté onion; add tomatoes and broth. Simmer until tomatoes are soft. Blend with fresh basil.

6. Quinoa and Chickpea Salad:

Description: A hearty salad with quinoa, chickpeas, colorful vegetables, and a light lemon dressing.

Benefits: Plant-based protein from quinoa and chickpeas; fiber and vitamins from vegetables.

Ingredients:

Quinoa, cooked

Chickpeas, drained and rinsed

Bell peppers, cucumber, cherry tomatoes, diced

Lemon dressing (low-sodium)

Preparation:

Combine quinoa, chickpeas, and diced vegetables. Drizzle with low-sodium lemon dressing.

7. **Chicken and Vegetable Soup:**

Description: A nourishing soup with lean chicken, a variety of vegetables, and fragrant herbs.

Benefits: Lean protein from chicken; vitamins and minerals from vegetables.

Ingredients:

Chicken breast, shredded

Carrots, celery, and potatoes, diced

Low-sodium chicken broth

Fresh thyme, rosemary

Preparation:

Cook chicken; add diced vegetables and broth. Simmer until vegetables are tender. Season with fresh thyme and rosemary.

8. **Spinach and Strawberry Salad:**

Description: A delightful salad with fresh spinach, juicy strawberries, almonds, and a balsamic vinaigrette.

Benefits: Iron and vitamins from spinach; antioxidants from strawberries.

Ingredients:

Fresh spinach leaves

Strawberries, sliced

Almonds, sliced

Balsamic vinaigrette (low-sodium)

Preparation:

Toss spinach, strawberries, and almonds. Drizzle with low-sodium balsamic vinaigrette.

8. Lentil Soup:

Description: Hearty lentil soup with carrots, celery, and onions, seasoned with cumin and coriander.

Benefits: Plant-based protein, fiber, and essential nutrients.

Ingredients:

Lentils

Carrots, celery, and onions, chopped

Low-sodium vegetable broth

Ground cumin, coriander

Preparation:

Cook lentils; add diced vegetables, broth, cumin, and coriander. Simmer until vegetables are tender.

9. Cucumber Avocado Gazpacho:

Description: A refreshing cold soup with cucumber, avocado, and a hint of lime.

Benefits: Hydration from cucumber; healthy fats from avocado.

Ingredients:

Cucumber, peeled and diced

Avocado, diced

Low-sodium vegetable broth

Lime juice

Preparation:

Blend cucumber, avocado, and broth until smooth. Stir in lime juice and chill before serving.

10. Chickpea and Vegetable Soup:

Description: A wholesome soup with chickpeas, tomatoes, carrots, and kale, seasoned with garlic and thyme.

Benefits: Plant-based protein, vitamins, and minerals.

Ingredients:

Chickpeas, cooked

Tomatoes, diced

Carrots, sliced

Kale, chopped

Low-sodium vegetable broth

Garlic, minced

Fresh thyme

Preparation:

Sauté garlic; add tomatoes, carrots, kale, chickpeas, and broth. Simmer until vegetables are tender. Season with fresh thyme.

12. Asian-Inspired Quinoa Salad:

Description: A vibrant quinoa salad with edamame, colorful bell peppers, and a ginger-soy dressing.

Benefits: Plant-based protein from quinoa and edamame; antioxidants from bell peppers.

Ingredients:

Quinoa, cooked

Edamame, shelled

Bell peppers (various colors), diced

Green onions, sliced

Ginger-soy dressing (low-sodium)

Preparation: Combine cooked quinoa, edamame, bell peppers, and green onions. Drizzle with low-sodium ginger-soy dressing.

13. Roasted Red Pepper and Tomato Soup:

Description: A velvety soup with roasted red peppers, tomatoes, and a touch of basil.

Benefits: Lycopene from tomatoes; low in fat and sodium.

Ingredients:

Roasted red peppers, diced

Tomatoes, chopped

Onion, chopped

Low-sodium vegetable broth

Fresh basil leaves

Preparation:

Sauté onion; add roasted red peppers, tomatoes, and broth. Simmer until vegetables are soft. Blend with fresh basil.

14. Mango Avocado Quinoa Salad:

Description: A tropical salad with quinoa, ripe mango, creamy avocado, and a cilantro-lime dressing.

Benefits: Healthy fats from avocado; vitamins and fiber from mango.

Ingredients:

Quinoa, cooked

Ripe mango, diced

Avocado, sliced

Cilantro-lime dressing (low-sodium)

Preparation:

Mix cooked quinoa with diced mango and sliced avocado. Drizzle with low-sodium cilantro-lime dressing.

15. Black Bean and Vegetable Chili:

Description: A hearty chili with black beans, tomatoes, bell peppers, and spices for a flavorful meal.

Benefits: Plant-based protein, fiber, and a variety of vegetables.

Ingredients:

Black beans, cooked

Tomatoes, diced, Bell peppers (various colors), chopped

Onion, diced, Chili powder, cumin, paprika

Low-sodium vegetable broth

Preparation:

Sauté onion; add tomatoes, bell peppers, black beans, and broth. Season with chili powder, cumin, and paprika. Simmer until vegetables are tender.

CHAPTER 5: HEART FRIENDLY DESERTS

1. Berry Parfait with Greek Yogurt:

Description: A refreshing parfait with layers of mixed berries and low-fat Greek yogurt.

Benefits: Antioxidants from berries; protein and probiotics from Greek yogurt.

Ingredients:

Mixed berries (strawberries, blueberries, raspberries)

Low-fat Greek yogurt

Honey (optional)

Preparation:

Layer mixed berries with Greek yogurt. Drizzle with honey if desired.

2. Dark Chocolate-Dipped Strawberries:

Description: Juicy strawberries dipped in dark chocolate for a satisfying yet heart-healthy treat.

Benefits: Antioxidants from dark chocolate; vitamins from strawberries.

Ingredients:

Fresh strawberries

Dark chocolate (70% cocoa or higher)

Preparation:

Melt dark chocolate; dip strawberries. Allow to set on parchment paper.

3. Baked Apples with Cinnamon:

Description: Baked apples sprinkled with cinnamon for a warm and comforting dessert.

Benefits: Fiber from apples; cinnamon for flavor without added sugar.

Ingredients:

Apples, cored and sliced

Cinnamon

Preparation:

Arrange apple slices in a baking dish; sprinkle with cinnamon. Bake until tender.

4. Chia Seed Pudding with Mango:

Description: Chia seed pudding with the sweetness of ripe mango.

Benefits: Omega-3s from chia seeds; vitamins and fiber from mango.

Ingredients:

Chia seeds

Almond milk

Ripe mango, diced

Preparation:

Mix chia seeds with almond milk; refrigerate until pudding-like consistency. Top with diced mango.

5. Frozen Banana Bites:

Description: Frozen banana slices dipped in a thin layer of yogurt for a cool and satisfying dessert.

Benefits: Potassium from bananas; probiotics from yogurt.

Ingredients:

Bananas, sliced

Low-fat yogurt

Preparation:

Dip banana slices in yogurt; freeze until solid.

6. Cinnamon Baked Pears:

Description: Baked pears with a sprinkle of cinnamon for a simple and flavorful dessert.

Benefits: Fiber and vitamins from pears; cinnamon for natural sweetness.

Ingredients:

Pears, halved

Cinnamon

Preparation:

Place pear halves in a baking dish; sprinkle with cinnamon. Bake until tender.

7. Mixed Berry Sorbet:

Description: Homemade sorbet with a blend of mixed berries for a refreshing treat.

Benefits: Antioxidants from berries; no added sugars.

Ingredients:

Mixed berries (strawberries, blueberries, raspberries)

Lemon juice

Preparation:

Blend berries with lemon juice; freeze until firm.

7. Oatmeal Raisin Cookies (Low-Fat Version):

Description: Soft and chewy oatmeal raisin cookies with reduced fat content.

Benefits: Whole grains from oats; sweetness from raisins.

Ingredients:

Rolled oats

Whole wheat flour

Raisins

Unsweetened applesauce

Preparation:

Mix oats, whole wheat flour, raisins, and applesauce. Bake until golden.

8. Peach and Almond Yogurt Parfait:

Description: Parfait with layers of fresh peaches, almond slices, and low-fat yogurt.

Benefits: Vitamins from peaches; healthy fats from almonds.

Ingredients:

Fresh peaches, sliced

Almond slices

Low-fat yogurt

Preparation:

Layer peaches, almonds, and yogurt in a glass.

9. Raspberry Chia Jam:

Description: Homemade chia seed jam with the tartness of raspberries.

Benefits: Omega-3s from chia seeds; antioxidants from raspberries.

Ingredients:

Raspberries

Chia seeds

Lemon juice

Preparation:

Mash raspberries; mix with chia seeds and lemon juice. Refrigerate until jam-like consistency.

10. Baked Cinnamon Bananas:

Description: Bananas baked with a sprinkle of cinnamon for a quick and healthy dessert.

Benefits: Potassium from bananas; natural sweetness from cinnamon.

Ingredients:

Bananas, sliced

Cinnamon

Preparation:

Arrange banana slices on a baking sheet; sprinkle with cinnamon. Bake until golden.

11. Mango Sorbet with Mint:

Description: Sorbet made with ripe mangoes and a touch of fresh mint.

Benefits: Vitamins and fiber from mango; refreshing mint flavor.

Ingredients:

Ripe mango, diced

Fresh mint leaves

Lime juice

Preparation:

Blend mango with mint and lime juice; freeze until firm.

12. Pumpkin Spice Baked Apples:

Description: Baked apples with a pumpkin spice twist for a cozy fall-inspired dessert.

Benefits: Fiber from apples; warming spices.

Ingredients:

Apples, cored and sliced

Pumpkin spice mix

Preparation:

Toss apple slices with pumpkin spice; bake until tender.

14. Coconut Chia Pudding with Pineapple:

Description: Chia seed pudding with coconut milk and chunks of sweet pineapple.

Benefits: Omega-3s from chia seeds; tropical sweetness from pineapple.

Ingredients:

Chia seeds

Coconut milk

Fresh pineapple, diced

Preparation:

Mix chia seeds with coconut milk; refrigerate until pudding-like consistency. Top with diced pineapple.

16. Blueberry Yogurt Popsicles:

Description: Homemade popsicles with a blend of blueberries and low-fat yogurt.

Benefits: Antioxidants from blueberries; probiotics from yogurt.

Ingredients:

Blueberries

Low-fat yogurt

Honey (optional)

Preparation:

Blend blueberries with yogurt; pour into popsicle molds. Freeze until solid.

CHAPTER 6: NOURISHING DINNER FOR HEART HEALTH

1. Grilled Lemon Herb Chicken:

Description: Tender grilled chicken marinated in a flavorful blend of lemon and herbs.

Benefits: Lean protein from chicken; refreshing citrus and herbs.

Ingredients:

Chicken breast

Lemon juice

Fresh herbs (rosemary, thyme)

Garlic, minced

Preparation:

Marinate chicken in lemon juice, herbs, and garlic. Grill until cooked through.

2. Salmon with Dill Sauce:

Description: Baked or grilled salmon topped with a light dill sauce.

Benefits: Omega-3 fatty acids from salmon; fresh flavor from dill.

Ingredients:

Salmon fillets

Fresh dill, chopped

Greek yogurt (low-fat)

Lemon juice

Preparation:

Bake or grill salmon; top with a mixture of chopped dill, Greek yogurt, and lemon juice.

3. Quinoa and Black Bean Stuffed Peppers:

Description: Colorful bell peppers stuffed with a nutritious mix of quinoa, black beans, and vegetables.

Benefits: Plant-based protein from quinoa and beans; fiber and vitamins from vegetables.

Ingredients:

Bell peppers, halved

Quinoa, cooked

Black beans, drained and rinsed

Tomatoes, corn, onions, diced

Preparation:

Mix cooked quinoa, black beans, and diced vegetables. Fill bell pepper halves and bake.

4. **Lemon Garlic Shrimp Stir-Fry:**

Description: Quick and tasty shrimp stir-fry with a zesty lemon and garlic sauce.

Benefits: Low in fat; lean protein from shrimp; citrusy and savory flavors.

Ingredients:

Shrimp, peeled and deveined

Broccoli, bell peppers, snap peas, sliced

Lemon juice

Garlic, minced

Preparation:

Stir-fry shrimp and vegetables in a wok with lemon juice and minced garlic until cooked.

5. Vegetarian Chickpea and Spinach Curry:

Description: Hearty curry with chickpeas, spinach, and aromatic spices.

Benefits: Plant-based protein from chickpeas; iron and vitamins from spinach.

Ingredients:

Chickpeas, cooked

Spinach

Tomatoes, onions, garlic, diced

Curry spices (turmeric, cumin, coriander)

Preparation:

Sauté onions and garlic; add tomatoes, chickpeas, spinach, and curry spices. Simmer until spinach wilts.

6. Turkey and Vegetable Skewers:

Description: Grilled turkey skewers with a medley of colorful vegetables.

Benefits: Lean protein from turkey; antioxidants from vegetables.

Ingredients:

Turkey breast, cubed

Bell peppers, cherry tomatoes, onions, sliced

Olive oil, herbs

Preparation:

Thread turkey and vegetables onto skewers. Grill until turkey is cooked.

7. Mushroom and Spinach Stuffed Chicken Breast:

Description: Chicken breasts stuffed with a flavorful mixture of mushrooms and spinach.

Benefits: Lean protein from chicken; vitamins and minerals from mushrooms and spinach.

Ingredients:

Chicken breast

Mushrooms, spinach, garlic, chopped

Low-fat mozzarella cheese

Preparation:

Sauté mushrooms, spinach, and garlic. Stuff the mixture into a pocket in the chicken breast. Bake until chicken is cooked. Top with a sprinkle of low-fat mozzarella.

8. Eggplant and Tomato Bake:

Description: Baked eggplant and tomato slices seasoned with herbs for a savory side or main dish.

Benefits: Low in fat; antioxidants from eggplant and tomatoes.

Ingredients:

Eggplant, tomatoes, sliced

Olive oil, garlic, herbs

Preparation:

Arrange alternating slices of eggplant and tomatoes in a baking dish. Drizzle with olive oil and sprinkle with minced garlic and herbs. Bake until tender.

8. Cauliflower and Chickpea Curry:

Description: A flavorful curry with cauliflower, chickpeas, and a blend of spices.

Benefits: Plant-based protein from chickpeas; vitamins and fiber from cauliflower.

Ingredients:

Cauliflower florets

Chickpeas, cooked

Tomatoes, onions, garlic, diced

Curry spices (cumin, coriander, turmeric)

Preparation:

Sauté onions and garlic; add tomatoes, chickpeas, cauliflower, and curry spices. Simmer until cauliflower is tender.

10. Spinach and Feta Stuffed Turkey Burgers:

Description: Turkey burgers filled with a mixture of spinach and feta for added flavor.

Benefits: Lean protein from turkey; iron and vitamins from spinach; flavor from feta.

Ingredients:

Ground turkey

Spinach, feta cheese, garlic, chopped

Preparation:

Mix ground turkey with chopped spinach, feta, and garlic. Form into patties and grill until cooked.

11. Sweet Potato and Lentil Soup:

Description: Hearty soup with sweet potatoes, lentils, and aromatic spices.

Benefits: Fiber and vitamins from sweet potatoes and lentils; warming spices.

Ingredients:

Sweet potatoes, lentils, onions, garlic, diced

Low-sodium vegetable broth

Cumin, coriander, paprika

Preparation:

Sauté onions and garlic; add sweet potatoes, lentils, broth, and spices. Simmer until sweet potatoes and lentils are tender.

12. Baked Lemon Herb Cod:

Description: Cod fillets baked with a zesty lemon and herb marinade.

Benefits: Lean protein from cod; citrusy and herby flavors.

Ingredients:

Cod fillets

Lemon juice

Fresh herbs (parsley, dill)

Garlic, minced

Preparation:

Marinate cod in lemon juice, herbs, and garlic. Bake until cooked through.

13. Black Bean and Vegetable Stir-Fry:

Description: Quick and colorful stir-fry with black beans, a variety of vegetables, and a low-sodium sauce.

Benefits: Plant-based protein from black beans; vitamins and fiber from vegetables.

Ingredients:

Black beans, cooked

Broccoli, bell peppers, carrots, sliced

Low-sodium stir-fry sauce

Preparation:

Stir-fry vegetables and black beans with a low-sodium stir-fry sauce until tender.

14. Tofu and Vegetable Skillet:

Description: Tofu stir-fry with a mix of colorful vegetables in a light soy and ginger sauce.

Benefits: Plant-based protein from tofu; antioxidants from vegetables.

Ingredients:

Extra-firm tofu, cubed

Broccoli, bell peppers, snap peas, sliced

Low-sodium soy sauce, ginger

Preparation:

Sauté tofu and vegetables with low-sodium soy sauce and ginger until heated through.

15. Cilantro Lime Shrimp Tacos:

Description: Flavorful cilantro lime shrimp served in whole-grain tortillas with fresh salsa.

Benefits: Lean protein from shrimp; whole grains from tortillas; freshness from salsa.

Ingredients:

Shrimp, peeled and deveined

Whole-grain tortillas

Fresh salsa (tomatoes, onions, cilantro, lime juice)

Preparation:

Sauté shrimp with cilantro and lime juice. Serve in whole-grain tortillas with fresh salsa.

CHAPTER 7: BEVERAGES FOR HYDRATION

1. Green Tea Citrus Cooler:

Description: Refreshing green tea infused with citrus fruits for a hydrating and antioxidant-rich beverage.

Benefits: Antioxidants from green tea; vitamin C from citrus fruits.

Ingredients:

Green tea bags

Lemon and orange slices

Mint leaves

Preparation:

Brew green tea; let it cool. Add citrus slices and mint leaves before serving over ice.

2. Hibiscus Berry Iced Tea:

Description: Hibiscus tea blended with mixed berries for a vibrant and heart-healthy iced tea.

Benefits: Hibiscus may help lower blood pressure; antioxidants from berries.

Ingredients:

Hibiscus tea bags

Mixed berries (strawberries, blueberries, raspberries)

Honey (optional)

Preparation:

Brew hibiscus tea; let it cool. Blend with mixed berries and sweeten with honey if desired. Serve over ice.

3. Cucumber Mint Infused Water:

Description: Light and refreshing water infused with cucumber slices and fresh mint.

Benefits: Hydration; cooling properties of cucumber; digestion aid from mint.

Ingredients:

Cucumber, thinly sliced

Fresh mint leaves

Preparation:

Combine cucumber slices and mint leaves in a pitcher of water. Let it infuse in the refrigerator before serving.

4. Berry Blast Smoothie:

Description: A smoothie packed with mixed berries, yogurt, and a splash of almond milk.

Benefits: Antioxidants from berries; probiotics from yogurt.

Ingredients:

Mixed berries (strawberries, blueberries, raspberries)

Low-fat yogurt

Almond milk

Preparation:

Blend mixed berries, yogurt, and almond milk until smooth. Serve chilled.

5. Golden Turmeric Latte:

Description: A warm and soothing latte with turmeric, known for its anti-inflammatory properties.

Benefits: Anti-inflammatory effects of turmeric.

Ingredients:

Turmeric powder

Almond milk

Cinnamon, ginger (optional)

Honey (optional)

Preparation:

Heat almond milk with turmeric, cinnamon, and ginger. Sweeten with honey if desired.

6. Watermelon Basil Lemonade:

Description: A summer-inspired lemonade with the sweetness of watermelon and a hint of basil.

Benefits: Hydration; vitamins from watermelon; refreshing basil flavor.

Ingredients:

Watermelon, blended

Lemon juice

Fresh basil leaves

Honey (optional)

Preparation:

Blend watermelon and strain to extract juice. Mix with lemon juice, fresh basil, and sweeten with honey if desired. Serve over ice.

7. Pineapple Coconut Smoothie:

Description: A tropical smoothie with the goodness of pineapple and the creaminess of coconut.

Benefits: Vitamins from pineapple; healthy fats from coconut.

Ingredients:

Pineapple chunks

Coconut milk (unsweetened)

Greek yogurt (low-fat)

Preparation:

Blend pineapple, coconut milk, and Greek yogurt until smooth. Serve chilled.

8. Lemon Ginger Iced Herbal Tea:

Description: Iced herbal tea infused with the zing of lemon and the warmth of ginger.

Benefits: Digestive aid from ginger; vitamin C from lemon.

Ingredients:

Herbal tea bags (chamomile or peppermint)

Lemon slices

Fresh ginger, sliced

Preparation:

Brew herbal tea; let it cool. Add lemon slices and ginger before serving over ice.

9. Cranberry Pomegranate Spritzer:

Description: A bubbly and tangy spritzer with the flavors of cranberry and pomegranate.

Benefits: Antioxidants from cranberry and pomegranate; hydration.

Ingredients:

Cranberry juice (unsweetened)

Pomegranate juice (unsweetened)

Sparkling water

Preparation:

Mix equal parts cranberry and pomegranate juice. Top with sparkling water and ice.

10. Mango Mint Green Smoothie:

Description: A vibrant green smoothie with the tropical sweetness of mango and a hint of mint.

Benefits: Vitamins from mango; refreshing mint flavor.

Ingredients:

Mango chunks

Spinach leaves

Mint leaves

Green tea (unsweetened)

Preparation:

Blend mango, spinach, mint, and green tea until smooth. Serve chilled.

11. Blueberry Lavender Lemonade:

Description: Lemonade infused with blueberries and a touch of calming lavender.

Benefits: Antioxidants from blueberries; calming effects of lavender.

Ingredients:

Blueberries

Lemon juice

Lavender syrup (made with dried lavender and honey)

Preparation:

Blend blueberries and strain to extract juice. Mix with lemon juice and lavender syrup. Serve over ice.

12. Peach Basil Iced Tea:

Description: Iced tea with the sweetness of peaches and a hint of basil for a unique twist.

Benefits: Antioxidants from tea; vitamins from peaches; refreshing basil flavor.

Ingredients:

Peach slices

Basil leaves

Black or green tea bags

Preparation:

Brew tea; let it cool. Add peach slices and basil leaves before serving over ice.

13. Cherry Almond Smoothie:

Description: A creamy smoothie with the rich flavor of cherries and a hint of almond.

Benefits: Antioxidants from cherries; healthy fats from almond.

Ingredients:

Cherries (fresh or frozen)

Almond milk

Greek yogurt (low-fat)

Preparation:

Blend cherries, almond milk, and Greek yogurt until smooth. Serve chilled.

14. Apple Cinnamon Spice Infused Water:

Description: Infused water with the classic combination of apple and cinnamon.

Benefits: Hydration; antioxidants from apples; warming spices.

Ingredients:

Apple slices

Cinnamon sticks

Preparation:

Combine apple slices and cinnamon sticks in a pitcher of water. Let it infuse before serving.

14. Carrot Ginger Turmeric Juice:

Description: A vibrant juice with the earthy flavors of carrot, the warmth of ginger, and the anti-inflammatory properties of turmeric.

Benefits: Vitamins from carrot; anti-inflammatory effects of turmeric; digestive aid from ginger.

Ingredients:

Carrots

Fresh ginger

Turmeric root

Preparation:

Juice carrots, ginger, and turmeric. Serve over ice.

CHAPTER 8: SNACKS AND APPETIZERS

1. Vegetable Crudité with Greek Yogurt Dip:

Description: Crisp and colorful vegetable sticks served with a light Greek yogurt dip.

Benefits: Fiber and vitamins from vegetables; protein and probiotics from Greek yogurt.

Ingredients:

Carrot, cucumber, bell pepper sticks

Greek yogurt (low-fat)

Lemon juice, dill (optional)

Preparation:

Arrange vegetable sticks on a plate. Mix Greek yogurt with lemon juice and dill for dipping.

2. Whole Grain Pita Chips with Hummus:

Description: Baked whole grain pita chips served with a flavorful and low-sodium hummus.

Benefits: Whole grains from pita; plant-based protein and fiber from hummus.

Ingredients:

Whole grain pita bread

Chickpeas, tahini, garlic, lemon juice

Preparation:

Cut pita bread into triangles, bake until crisp. Blend chickpeas, tahini, garlic, and lemon juice for hummus.

3. Cucumber Avocado Salsa:

Description: A refreshing salsa with cucumber, avocado, and tomatoes, perfect with whole-grain chips.

Benefits: Healthy fats from avocado; vitamins from vegetables.

Ingredients:

Cucumber, avocado, tomatoes, diced

Red onion, cilantro, lime juice

Preparation:

Mix diced cucumber, avocado, tomatoes, red onion, cilantro, and lime juice.

4. **Edamame and Sea Salt:**

Description: Steamed edamame sprinkled with a touch of sea salt for a protein-packed snack.

Benefits: Plant-based protein from edamame; minimal sodium.

Ingredients:

Edamame (in pods)

Sea salt

Preparation:

Steam edamame pods until tender. Sprinkle with sea salt before serving.

5. Baked Sweet Potato Fries:

Description: Oven-baked sweet potato fries seasoned with herbs for a nutritious alternative to regular fries.

Benefits: Vitamins and fiber from sweet potatoes; low in fat.

Ingredients:

Sweet potatoes, cut into fries

Olive oil, rosemary, thyme

Preparation:

Toss sweet potato fries with olive oil and herbs. Bake until golden.

6. Caprese Skewers:

Description: Skewers with cherry tomatoes, fresh mozzarella, and basil drizzled with balsamic glaze.

Benefits: Antioxidants from tomatoes; calcium from mozzarella; freshness from basil.

Ingredients:

Cherry tomatoes

Fresh mozzarella balls

Fresh basil leaves

Balsamic glaze

Preparation:

Thread tomatoes, mozzarella, and basil onto skewers. Drizzle with balsamic glaze.

7. Roasted Chickpeas:

Description: Crispy roasted chickpeas seasoned with a mix of spices for a flavorful snack.

Benefits: Plant-based protein and fiber from chickpeas; low in fat.

Ingredients:

Canned chickpeas, drained and dried

Olive oil, cumin, paprika, garlic powder

Preparation:

Toss dried chickpeas with olive oil and spices. Roast until crunchy.

8. Guacamole with Veggie Sticks:

Description: Homemade guacamole served with carrot and cucumber sticks.

Benefits: Healthy fats from avocado; vitamins from vegetables.

Ingredients:

Avocado, tomatoes, onions, cilantro, lime juice

Carrot and cucumber sticks

Preparation:

Mash avocado; mix with diced tomatoes, onions, cilantro, and lime juice. Serve with veggie sticks.

9. Mango Salsa with Baked Tortilla Chips:

Description: A sweet and spicy mango salsa paired with baked whole-grain tortilla chips.

Benefits: Vitamins from mango; whole grains from tortilla chips.

Ingredients:

Mango, red onion, jalapeño, cilantro

Whole-grain tortilla wraps

Preparation:

Dice mango, red onion, jalapeño, and cilantro for salsa. Cut tortillas into triangles, bake until crisp.

10. Greek Yogurt and Berry Parfait:

Description: Layers of low-fat Greek yogurt, mixed berries, and a sprinkle of granola.

Benefits: Protein and probiotics from Greek yogurt; antioxidants from berries.

Ingredients:

Low-fat Greek yogurt

Mixed berries (strawberries, blueberries)

Granola (low-sugar)

Preparation:

Layer Greek yogurt, berries, and granola in a glass.

11. Spicy Baked Zucchini Chips:

Description: Zucchini slices seasoned with spices and baked until crispy.

Benefits: Low in fat; vitamins and fiber from zucchini.

Ingredients:

Zucchini, thinly sliced

Olive oil, chili powder, cumin, garlic powder

Preparation:

Toss zucchini slices with olive oil and spices. Bake until crispy.

12. Chia Seed Pudding with Fresh Berries:

Description: Chia seed pudding made with almond milk, topped with fresh berries.

Benefits: Omega-3 fatty acids from chia seeds; antioxidants from berries.

Ingredients:

Chia seeds

Almond milk (unsweetened)

Mixed berries

Preparation:

Mix chia seeds with almond milk; refrigerate until pudding consistency. Top with fresh berries before serving.

13. Stuffed Mini Bell Peppers:

Description: Mini bell peppers stuffed with a mix of hummus or cottage cheese and herbs.

Benefits: Fiber and vitamins from bell peppers; protein from hummus or cottage cheese.

Ingredients:

Mini bell peppers

Hummus or low-fat cottage cheese

Herbs (chives, parsley)

Preparation:

Cut bell peppers in half; fill with hummus or cottage cheese. Garnish with herbs.

14. Turkey and Vegetable Lettuce Wraps:

Description: Lettuce wraps filled with lean ground turkey and a medley of vegetables.

Benefits: Lean protein from turkey; vitamins and fiber from vegetables.

Ingredients:

Ground turkey

Lettuce leaves (butter or iceberg)

Bell peppers, onions, carrots, sliced

Preparation:

Sauté ground turkey and vegetables. Spoon into lettuce leaves.

15. Apple and Almond Butter Sandwiches:

Description: Slices of apple sandwiched with almond butter for a satisfying and nutritious snack.

Benefits: Healthy fats from almond butter; vitamins and fiber from apples.

Ingredients:

Apple, sliced

Almond butter (unsweetened)

Preparation:

Spread almond butter between apple slices to create sandwiches.

CONCLUSION

This Congestive *Heart Failure Cookbook* is more than just a collection of recipes, it's a comprehensive guide to a heart-healthy lifestyle crafted with care and consideration for those navigating the challenges of congestive heart failure. As we've explored the diverse and flavorful array of low-fat, low-sodium recipes within these pages, the overarching goal has been to empower individuals to take control of their health without sacrificing the joy of eating.

The benefits of embracing the recipes in this cookbook extend far beyond the pleasure of savoring delicious meals. By adopting the principles of a low-fat and low-sodium diet, individuals with congestive heart failure can experience a positive impact on their overall well-being. The carefully curated recipes prioritize nutrient-rich ingredients, offering essential vitamins, minerals, and antioxidants crucial for heart health.

This cookbook serves as a practical tool for managing blood pressure, reducing sodium intake, and improving heart function. The thoughtfully crafted recipes do not only support cardiovascular health but also cater to the diverse tastes and preferences of individuals, proving that maintaining a heart-healthy diet can be a flavorsome and enjoyable journey.

Ultimately, this cookbook is a celebration of the belief that wholesome, heart-healthy eating is not a restriction but an opportunity. It's an opportunity to savor the joy of delicious meals, to appreciate the vibrant colors and flavors that nature provides, and most importantly, to embrace a lifestyle that promotes a healthier, happier heart.

7-WEEK MEAL PLANNING

Meal Planner

Date:

Monday
BREAKFAST

LUNCH

DINNER

DESSERTS

Tuesday
BREAKFAST

LUNCH

DINNER

DESSERTS

Wednesday
BREAKFAST

LUNCH

DINNER

DESSERTS

Thursday
BREAKFAST

LUNCH

DINNER

DESSERTS

Friday
BREAKFAST

LUNCH

DINNER

DESSERTS

Saturday
BREAKFAST

LUNCH

DINNER

DESSERTS

Sunday
BREAKFAST

LUNCH

DINNER

DESSERTS

NOTES:

WEEK 2

Meal Planner

Date:

Monday
BREAKFAST

LUNCH

DINNER

DESSERTS

Tuesday
BREAKFAST

LUNCH

DINNER

DESSERTS

Wednesday
BREAKFAST

LUNCH

DINNER

DESSERTS

Thursday
BREAKFAST

LUNCH

DINNER

DESSERTS

Friday
BREAKFAST

LUNCH

DINNER

DESSERTS

Saturday
BREAKFAST

LUNCH

DINNER

DESSERTS

Sunday
BREAKFAST

LUNCH

DINNER

DESSERTS

NOTES:

WEEK 3

Meal Planner

Date:

Monday
BREAKFAST

LUNCH

DINNER

DESSERTS

Tuesday
BREAKFAST

LUNCH

DINNER

DESSERTS

Wednesday
BREAKFAST

LUNCH

DINNER

DESSERTS

Thursday
BREAKFAST

LUNCH

DINNER

DESSERTS

Friday
BREAKFAST

LUNCH

DINNER

DESSERTS

Saturday
BREAKFAST

LUNCH

DINNER

DESSERTS

Sunday
BREAKFAST

LUNCH

DINNER

DESSERTS

NOTES:

WEEK 4

Meal Planner

Date:

Monday
BREAKFAST

LUNCH

DINNER

DESSERTS

Tuesday
BREAKFAST

LUNCH

DINNER

DESSERTS

Wednesday
BREAKFAST

LUNCH

DINNER

DESSERTS

Thursday
BREAKFAST

LUNCH

DINNER

DESSERTS

Friday
BREAKFAST

LUNCH

DINNER

DESSERTS

Saturday
BREAKFAST

LUNCH

DINNER

DESSERTS

Sunday
BREAKFAST

LUNCH

DINNER

DESSERTS

NOTES:

WEEK 5

Meal Planner

Date:

Monday
BREAKFAST

LUNCH

DINNER

DESSERTS

Tuesday
BREAKFAST

LUNCH

DINNER

DESSERTS

Wednesday
BREAKFAST

LUNCH

DINNER

DESSERTS

Thursday
BREAKFAST

LUNCH

DINNER

DESSERTS

Friday
BREAKFAST

LUNCH

DINNER

DESSERTS

Saturday
BREAKFAST

LUNCH

DINNER

DESSERTS

Sunday
BREAKFAST

LUNCH

DINNER

DESSERTS

NOTES:

WEEK 6

Meal Planner

Date:

Monday
BREAKFAST

LUNCH

DINNER

DESSERTS

Tuesday
BREAKFAST

LUNCH

DINNER

DESSERTS

Wednesday
BREAKFAST

LUNCH

DINNER

DESSERTS

Thursday
BREAKFAST

LUNCH

DINNER

DESSERTS

Friday
BREAKFAST

LUNCH

DINNER

DESSERTS

Saturday
BREAKFAST

LUNCH

DINNER

DESSERTS

Sunday
BREAKFAST

LUNCH

DINNER

DESSERTS

NOTES:

WEEK 7

Meal Planner

Date:

Monday
BREAKFAST

LUNCH

DINNER

DESSERTS

Tuesday
BREAKFAST

LUNCH

DINNER

DESSERTS

Wednesday
BREAKFAST

LUNCH

DINNER

DESSERTS

Thursday
BREAKFAST

LUNCH

DINNER

DESSERTS

Friday
BREAKFAST

LUNCH

DINNER

DESSERTS

Saturday
BREAKFAST

LUNCH

DINNER

DESSERTS

Sunday
BREAKFAST

LUNCH

DINNER

DESSERTS

NOTES:

Manufactured by Amazon.ca
Acheson, AB